Vegan Diet

30 Days of Vegan Recipes and Meal Plans to
Increase Your Health and Energy

(Weight Loss and Leading a Healthy Lifestyle)

Fred Dowd

Published by Robert Satterfield Publishing House

© **Fred Dowd**

All Rights Reserved

Vegan Diet: 30 Days of Vegan Recipes and Meal Plans to Increase Your Health and Energy (Weight Loss and Leading a Healthy Lifestyle)

ISBN 978-1-989682-99-9

All rights reserved. No part of this guide may be reproduced in any form without permission in writing from the publisher except in the case of brief quotations embodied in critical articles or reviews.

Legal & Disclaimer

The information contained in this book is not designed to replace or take the place of any form of medicine or professional medical advice. The information in this book has been provided for educational and entertainment purposes only.

The information contained in this book has been compiled from sources deemed reliable, and it is accurate to the best of the Author's knowledge; however, the Author cannot guarantee its accuracy and validity and cannot be held liable for any errors or omissions. Changes are periodically made to this book. You must consult your doctor or get professional medical advice before using any of the suggested remedies, techniques, or information in this book.

TABLE OF CONTENT

Part 1 1

Introduction... 2

Chapter 1: Why Vegan – And What Does That Mean, Anyway? 5

Chapter 2: Food – Is It Destroying Or Creating Your Health And Energy Levels?... 13

Chapter 3: Go Cold Turkey Or Ease Into This?.................... 34

Chapter 4: Recipes – Cooked Transitioning For Health 42

Recipes 44

Chapter 5: Recipes – Raw, Living, Energizing And Delicious 59

Cherry Tomato Beet Top Dressing....................................... 61

Yellow Bell Pepper Mango Dressing 62

Cashew Cheese.. 64

No-Bean Bean Dip 65

Power Pate 67

3 Ways To Enjoy Pate 69

Conclusion 71

Part 2 74

Introduction... 75

Delicious Vegan Recipes... 76

Sweet Tasting Carrot Risotto	76
Savory Blueberry Scones	79
Streusel Topped Coffee Cake	81
Orange Style French Toast	83
Vegan Style Banana Bread	85
Matzo Meal Pancakes	87
Sticky Cinnamon Buns	89
Vegan Style Pumpkin Spiced Pancakes	91
Vegan Style Chicken Alfredo Lasagna Rolls	93
Vegan Style Cheese Stuffed Burger	95
Easy Vegan Mac And Cheese	97
Healthy Avocado Pesto Pasta	98
Classic Caesar Salad	100
Homemade Creamy Tomato Soup	103
Hawaiian Style Sloppy Joes	105
Winter Style White Bean Salad	108
Hearty Portobello Mushroom Burgers	110
Mongolian Style Bbq Seitan	112
Tasty Mushroom Stroganoff	114
Tempeh Chimichurri	116
Classic Penne Marinara	118
Hearty Shepherd's Pie	120

Decadent Chocolate And Strawberry Shortcake Cupcakes 123

Decadent Peanut Butter Bonbons 126

Zesty Lemon Bars 128

Conclusion 130

About The Author 132

Part 1

Introduction

This is for those of you who have decided that your levels of health and energy may benefit from going vegan. There is enough scientific, factual and indisputable evidence – not to mention anecdotal success stories – to demonstrate to us that eating a diet of plant foods is good for us.

"Going Vegan" is not about adopting one of the hundreds of "diets" that are out there. It is simply a 21st-century trend in taking personal responsibility for your own health, vitality, energy levels and overall wellness. It is simply a decision to go back to nature and choose living, nutritious and health-giving foods – as Mother Nature provides them to us.

You can recreate natural health and wellness, virtually through food alone. I'm not making this up. I'm not just sharing my personal experience. The medical, scientific and academic communities have been studying the contribution of whole, fresh, natural fruit and vegetables, nuts and seeds to our body's health for decades. Agro food lobbyists don't want us to know how good raw, whole plant foods are for our health, because their paycheck comes from processing foods! However, more and more physicians are advising their patients to take charge of their own health improvement by going vegan to some degree.

If you're reading this book, you've either made a decision to go vegan based on your personal research – or a doctor in the know is pointing you down this path. Either way, I'll give you all the guidance you need to easily get started down the path to greater health and vitality by eating more plant foods. If you are like me, after a few weeks on such a plan, you will have energy to burn like never before! You will lose a few pounds … or many. Your "lab" numbers will improve, and you may just decide with your doctor that some of your medications are no longer needed. Maybe you will be moved to get out there and exercise a little bit more than usual... or just want to do it for the first time.

The science is clear. Anecdotal success stories abound. The healing that people are able to do is undeniable. Going vegan is good for your health, your energy, and your overall happiness. Happiness? Yes, I guarantee that when (and NOT if) you get your health back through delicious fresh food, you will definitely be happy about it!

Chapter 1: Why Vegan – and What Does that Mean, Anyway?

So, what does it mean to be vegetarian or a vegan?

Unfortunately, if you search for information to define a vegetarian or a vegan, not everyone agrees what these mean. Let's keep it very simple for our purposes.

"Veg" refers of course to vegetation or **plants**. A vegetarian gets nourishment **primarily**, but not only, from plant foods. A vegetarian may eat some dairy products, some eggs and very occasionally some fish. That's why we say their calories and nutrients comes **mostly** from plant foods.

A vegan gets nourishment **solely** from plant foods. A vegan will never eat any food from an animal source. Don't bother to ask a vegan if he eats fish or eggs! A fish is an animal; eggs are from and become animals. Don't bother to ask a vegan if he'd like some sour cream. Sour cream is a dairy product, and all dairy products come from animals, don't they?

Both vegetarians and vegans may cook some of their plant foods, and eat some of them raw. A vegan who prefers to eat only raw plant foods is called a raw foodist or a raw-food-vegan, and some jokingly call them uncooked vegans.

The serious adherents to either the all-raw vegan or the cooked vegan approach never, ever eat refined or processed foods (more on that later).

Now You

I will not be going very much into the benefits of going vegan because if you are reading this book, you have already discovered how going vegan might help you. My goal is to help you get started in this way of preparing and eating food.

Why are you going vegan? The answer is very important – whatever it is. Making any lifestyle change is tough, and it's even tougher when it comes to making changes in your food choices or kitchen routines. Because of that, you need to be motivated for yourself (and not for other individuals around you) or you'll go back to your old ways. So sit down right now and ask yourself why you choose to make this change. Or – why you **must** make this change. Write as many reasons as you can.

Most individuals are stuck like glue to their personal food choices and eating routines, and this is not because they have allergies leading them to avoid some foods! It is very often a question of the food not tasting pleasant to the individual, or its texture feeling unpleasant in the mouth. Some of us like hot and spicy foods, others of us enjoy sweetness and so on.

Some food choices arise for reasons the individual himself cannot pinpoint because they come from deep childhood experiences. It is just a long-ingrained habit. Be that as it may. If you are not vegan today, you need to face the fact that these changes will stir up some resistance!

Tips for Beating Off the Resistance

Yes, to resist change is human, so you need some strategies for dealing with it when it surges up and tells you to go grab that bag of chips or to just zip up to the takeout window and order a burger and fries.

#1: This is the top thing to pay attention to! It applies to raw vegans and cooked vegans alike. **Always have your go-bags, fridge and kitchen stocked** up with grab-and-eat raw fruit, fresh vegetables, nuts.

Have a supply of countertop grab-and-eat food like washed apples and pears in a kitchen counter basket, bananas to tuck into your carryall, backpack or go-bag. Fruit has sufficient calories to keep you going for hours when you eat enough of it.

Have raw nuts that you have prepacked in small Ziploc snack bags ready to go for you. I like to pretend that raw nuts are like chewing gum — I keep chewing and chewing to get all the nutritional goodness out of it before swallowing. The fat content can keep you going for hours, and I prefer to eat nuts early in the day for this reason.

In the summertime, seasonal tomatoes of any type are thirst-quenching go-to "snacks" between meals. Prewashed carrots, whether you cut them up or not, along with prewashed celery sticks are good grab-and-go foods that keep you hydrated and filled (because of the fiber content they all have) until you can sit for a full meal.

#2: Have an **eating plan** for a full week. Have an eating plan for social events outside your home. Again, this applies to both raw vegans and cooked vegans.

A big part of having an eating plan for a full week is that it also becomes your **shopping list**. Many vegans that I know go shopping a minimum of two times weekly — often to their farmer's market, but definitely to the local produce department of the grocer's.

- Don't let yourself run out of ingredients for your eating plan! When I know I can shop two or even three times weekly, I still have a full week's eating plan to work from. I keep the list in my go bag or wallet, so that when I do arrive at the market, I know exactly what I need to purchase.
- Most people know their social calendar for at least a week in advance. I realize spontaneity calls to us every once in a while! This is where you have an eating plan for social events, even for the weeks there are no social events on your calendar.
- It is your job to make this easy for your friends — not the reverse! I cannot tell you how many friends who have invited me to their homes for dinner, and then fretted about "what to feed me, the raw food vegan". Generally, when I arrive, I take them to their refrigerator and their countertop fruit basket, and I ask them to show me the

fruit and vegetables they have. When I tell them that's what I'll eat, some of them relax, but some still wring their hands with how to prepare those vegetables and fruits. When I tell them, "Just wash them and put them on a plate for me", that does get some laughter. KEEP IT EASY FOR THEM.

- If a social event involves a restaurant which is not strictly vegetarian or even vegan, remember that it is a restaurant. That means the kitchen is probably full of fruit and vegetables, even though the menu combines them with fish and meat, cheese and dairy products. Simply ask for this or that salad from the menu to be served without grated cheese or shaved ham! I have worked in restaurant kitchens, and I know that most professional cooks and chefs **enjoy it** when they get a customized order like that.

This said, don't be too hard on the waiter because he is not in the kitchen! Don't be that awful customer who questions the waiter on every last little ingredient of any dish. Honey, the waiter does not know! Stop asking. Don't be that awful customer who tries to rewrite the menu. KEEP IT SIMPLE. If you're hungry after a restaurant meal – go home and eat! No big deal.

Hopefully, in these pages, you will find not only a plan that suits you but easy (and sometimes quite familiar) recipes to help you slide into a vegan lifestyle.

Chapter 2: Food – Is It Destroying or Creating Your Health and Energy Levels?

If you are already mentally and physically healthy, eating plant foods will help to keep you that way. If you are healthy, but developing a tendency to gain and retain weight, eating plant foods will help you slim down at a healthy pace and maintain a healthy weight. If you are taking any mental health prescriptions, you can alleviate your need for them by increasing your RAW micronutrient intake (also known as nutrition from raw green and other colorful vegetables and fruit). If you have one or more physical illness diagnoses for which you are taking doctor prescribed medications, eating plant foods has been demonstrated to help get you back to a state of health and wellness. And, though I am not a doctor by any means, anecdotal success stories from many people able to drop their medications entirely due to eating vegan-style are too numerous to ignore.

Maybe you have a diagnosis that your doctor has assured you can be reversed by changing what you eat. The common diagnoses in this category (but not, by far, all of them!) include diabetes, high blood pressure and all heart-related (aka cardio-vascular) ailments, overweight (no matter how few or how many pounds), unhealthy cholesterol levels and most digestive or gastric disorders.

*All afflictions are **dramatically reduced or eliminated** by going vegan.*

This has been demonstrated, measured and proven time and again.

Speaking only of the United States here, our agricultural industry has very successfully created lots and lots of inexpensive food for us since the Second World War. However, big corporations (which I will not name, as this is easily the subject of a whole new book) have pushed that mandate and created GMO (genetically modified organisms) as our "new" seeds for foods. These are now producing food shown to be less healthy for us than Mother Nature's organic plants over the long term for the human being. Even GMO farmers are unhappy, since those seeds have lower yields than organic and heirloom seeds do, and so they earn less money.

I am assuming that you have already read up on some of the evidence supporting my statements, or in another way come to the conclusion that you're ready to resolve your health issues by going vegan.

Health-Sapping "Foods"

If you are re-creating lost health as a vegan, you will want to avoid GMO, refined and processed foods (and it is very easy these days). A good way to start avoiding GMO foods is to **stop eating anything containing wheat or corn**. This includes primarily any packaged, processed foods – because they are produced with some form of corn or wheat, regardless of what labels may state. In the US, we have habitually used packaged products as snack, breakfast or side dish foods in our diets. Stop it! This also naturally includes corn itself (even on the cob), all wheat-containing pasta products, all baked goods and bakery desserts. Aside from the raw corn itself, you can easily see that products containing wheat or corn are processed – and thus, as a vegan (as we have defined it here, and whether raw or cooked vegan) you will naturally avoid these foods anyway!

You are going to prefer all raw (organic, too – as much as you can find and afford them) fruits and vegetables, nuts, and seeds. I say to avoid refined and processed foods for a bunch of good reasons:

1. *Refined, processed foods include* **sugars and sweeteners** *of all kinds (most of them made in a factory, rather than from a plant from your garden), whether they come in paper bags or*

paper packets or in jars of liquid sweetness. You will be eating more fruit than ever before, including dried fruit such as dates or dried apricots, and using fruit to sweeten other dishes. You no longer need any of the sugars or sweeteners that are now in your cupboard. In fact, you never needed them – they have been destroying your health!

2. As you read on, you will notice that my recipes never use salt, not even the "good" organic or sea salts. Refined and processed foods are filled not only with those sugars I just mentioned but various forms of **salt and sodium**. Your body does not need these ingredients! Also, note that all raw plants including fruit contain some natural and healthy sodium – always in just the right amount for your body to process and benefit from. Plus, our bodies don't like the types of sodium used in processed foods! Our bodies are just toxic and

sick from the sodium we've been feeding it.
3. As you eat in restaurants, many of the ingredients of your meal are from processed food packages that the restaurant is simply reheating or presenting in a different way. All of those processed foods are high in sodium, sugars, and... let's say the word – fat! We have been trained like lab rats to believe that over-salted, over-sweetened and overly fatty or oily foods taste better. Your body has another viewpoint! As a new vegan, you will learn which plant foods contain fat, and it is the healthy, body-friendly version. While that doesn't give you a free pass to eat all you want of those fat-containing foods, you will learn how to make recipes including these healthy fat foods, so that you get plenty of health-producing fats in your diet.

All Vegans No-Go List

Here, listed below, are most of the "foods" you will no longer be eating as a vegan. If you have any of them in your kitchen or your pantry, pack it up, and carry it off to your local Food Bank – or give it to someone you know who really needs it because they're on a tight food budget:

- Meat, fish, eggs, dairy foods like creams and cheese
- Canned foods (in spite of claims, it is either filled with sodium, sweetening agents, fats – or just plain stripped of its nutritional value through overheating)
- Frozen processed foods, like frozen dinners, pizzas, premade burgers or frozen juices
- All the condiments in the door of your fridge, except olives or spices that come from plants
- Most of the condiments in your cupboard, especially "mixed" or blended condiments which do not list all ingredients, or which contain salt (and all spice bottles you have owned

for more than 6 months – yes, they "go bad")
- All food in crinkly soft packs, like Ramen noodles, chips, and snacks, or energy bars
- All food in boxes, like breakfast cereals, "minute" rice or potato flakes, bread crumbs, and croutons
- Wheat and corn containing processed foods
- Sweetening agents, like honey, agave nectar, white or brown sugar, artificial sweeteners and so on, including anything you add to coffee or tea like powdered milk or a processed creamer
- Sodas and **all** beverages in cans and bottles (except water for when you are on the go) including all liquor, however, "light" or high in alcohol.

Raw Vegans No-Go List

For those of you choosing raw vegan strategies, you *additionally* will no longer be buying or eating these foods, whether or not they are organic:

- Wheat or other types of flour, cornmeal, pasta and any other refined grains used in baking or other cooked dishes – YES, I am repeating myself. Toss 'em out!
- Rice, even brown
- Canned beans (because they are cooked, right?)
- Larger dried beans (like kidney beans) that are not sproutable and edible as sprouts due to incompatibility with our tummy's chemistry
- Bottled oils and coconut oil, even organic
- Caffeine from both tea and coffee

Think of all the cash you are going to be saving, by no longer purchasing ANY of these "foods"!!

Health Building Foods

If you are re-creating lost health, you will also have to get your head out of the sand and educate yourself with real scientific evidence. I know we get no factual food education in our schools, but with the Internet, it's very easy to educate yourself. Inspire yourself as well with Success Stories – YouTube is filled with meat-to-vegan or junk-food-to-raw-vegan transformation stories. Likewise, many long-time vegans give us excellent tips in their blogs and vlogs.

The Short Version

The short version of what to do? Eliminate from your kitchen and cupboards anything and everything you used to eat that is **NOT** in the following list. Becoming a vegan gets really simple when you grow a garden with, shop for and eat only:

- Fresh, raw fruit
- Dried fruit (like air-dried apricots, figs or dates)

- Fresh, raw vegetables of any color
- Dried vegetables (like sun-dried tomatoes)
- Raw nuts of any type – soaked for 2 hours and drained before consuming
- Raw seeds of any type – including their sprouted forms
- Sea vegetables (in other words, seaweeds)

See how easy it is to stock an all-vegan refrigerator? If you cannot buy it in the produce section of your grocery store, grow it in the back garden or find it at the farmer's market, it is probably not anything you will be eating as a vegan!

And to make it really easy for you here is a list of more detailed real food which you will be looking for, purchasing and experimenting with eating as a vegan. Let's look at this real food in terms of fat, sweet, and savory items. Or – in traditional terms – fat, fruit, vegetables.

FAT

The top raw and healthy fat-containing foods are delicious. Don't overdo these foods, just as you would never overdo oil out of a bottle, nor eat a huge fat-marbled steak three times a day in your pre-vegan days. This said, there is nothing wrong with an avocado a day, and a handful of olives or raw nuts that same day. Balance in all things!

Avocados

Olives (not the stuffed variety)

Raw nuts and seeds of all types, organic when you can find them (do not buy peanuts unless they are guaranteed organic – too many issues with them otherwise)

Chia and flax seeds

Chia and flaxseeds get their own shout-out, for two reasons. First, we don't sprout them. Second, they are not usually eaten on their own like the other types of fat foods but are nutritious ingredients in other dishes you prepare. Also, flaxseeds do your body absolutely no good (and also no harm, by the way) unless you crush or grind them. Use a coffee grinder or a dry Vitamix to do so at each use. Chia seeds do not need to be ground to benefit your body, but they can be if you wish.

Look at the raw recipe chapter for Basic Pudding to see one way to use Flax or Chia seeds. Or just toss them into any vegetable or fruit smoothie that you happen to be making. One last way that many vegans use these seeds is to toss them in a whole food salad, either in the dressing or just in the salad bowl.

SWEET

This includes all fresh fruit, naturally. This also includes naturally dried fruit, such as dates, raisins or apricots. Again, balance in all things, please – far too many vegans go overboard with fruit. Far too many all-raw vegans overuse dates (in my opinion) in their sweet-food concoctions and complex dessert recipes. Don't do it! Being a cooked vegan or a raw food vegan does not mean you get to cave into your sweet tooth morning, noon and night! Fresh fruit, eaten whole, provides half or more of your daily calories, yes. Dried fruit should be seen as a treat, much as chocolate or a baked dessert is seen as a treat for a disciplined non-vegan eater.

Buy fresh, seasonal fruit for your region of the world. There are dozens and hundreds of types of fruit on the planet, but here are some common ones to help you get started that you can get in **summertime** (depending on where you live, that can be from April through November):

- Apricots
- Bananas
- Pears
- Berries of all types – Blueberries, Blackberries, Raspberries and Strawberries
- Cantaloupe, Honeydew Melon, Watermelon

- Cherries
- Grapes
- Citrus fruit of all types – Lemons, Tangerines, Mandarin Oranges, Oranges, Grapefruit
- Apples
- Plums
- Peaches

No need to get exotic when you're starting out! Buy what you know. Buy what you like.

Supermarkets have tricked us into believing that apples, tomatoes and other fruit and vegetables are seasonal 12 months a year. Not true! They simply have a worldwide network of farmers and growers, and "chase" oranges and apples around the globe to bring them home to us all year.

If you want to truly find out what the seasonal fruit is for your area, go to the farmer's market. If every farmer is selling the same variety of fruit, you know that it is in season. So buy it! Eat lots of it!

Mother Nature made no mistake when it created seasonal fruits – because the nutritional content of the fruit is exactly what our body needs during that season. It boggles the mind how doing things according to nature brings back health and balance to our bodies!

SAVORY

The same goes for seasonal vegetables for your region of the world. Find out what they are, and buy them. Experiment with different preparations.

Purchase lots and lots of green leafy vegetables. Always have some in the fridge! Eat some at every meal! (I even add them to my fruit smoothies in the mornings). In summer, the green leafy vegetables will be tender leaf types of lettuces and so on. In winter, your green leafy vegetables will be of tougher varieties such as all the types of cabbages and kale that exist and so on.

Purchase the rest of your vegetables in a rainbow of bright colors. Mother Nature, yet again, shows us through color how differently colored vegetables contain different nutrients needed seasonally by our bodies. Trust seasonal vegetables.

Here are vegetables that you can get in **summertime** (depending on where you live, that can be from April through November):

- Cucumber
- Beets
- Bell Peppers – all colors
- Squash, zucchini
- Green beans
- Eggplant (for cooked vegans)
- Celery
- Snap peas
- Radishes
- Lettuces and leafy greens of all kinds
- Spicy peppers
- Tomatoes – all varieties and colors

It's not summertime? The farmer's market is a good indicator of what these seasonal vegetables are, and you can also question your neighborhood vegetable gardeners for the same information. Mother Nature, again, makes no mistakes in matching up seasonal produce with our bodies' energetic needs. Go with seasonality as much as you can for all of your vegetables.

By buying seasonal fruit and vegetables, you will also experience one other appreciable benefit: you will save money. Buying seasonal produce means that you buy it when there is a local bumper crop of these fruits and vegetables, and when there is a large crop the Law of Supply and Demand kicks in and you pay less.

The Vegan Kitchen

If you don't have "energy to burn" all day long right now (or any day, really), as a new vegan you can help change that. Just STOP:

- Microwaving any food (no, not even to warm it up)
- Buying anything at a fast food business
- Eating and preparing overcooked foods

You will need to get into new kitchen and food preparation routines. Maybe you need to ban trips to the restaurant or fast food take out window for a month until you are kick-started. Your health demands it. You deserve it.

If you have enjoyed cooking at home up until now, chances are you have all of the manual or electric appliances that will make becoming and remaining vegan enjoyable.

I surveyed a few vegan friends about this, and here are the manual tools, utensils or small appliances they all seem to use:

- Sharp kitchen knives, in two or three sizes, and a sharpening tool for them
- Cutting board

- Hand grater/slicer
- Apple corer/slicer
- Peeler
- Food processor, like a Cuisinart, for grinding/blending vegetables very easily without unwanted liquids, or for slicing/grating them
- Blender, the most popular being the Vitamix for its versatility, for smoothies and salad dressings – a stick blender works well, too
- Citrus press, whether manual or electric, for your lemons, oranges and so on
- Spiralizer, the most popular being the Poderno brand, for turning vegetables into fettuccine, angel hair or flat noodle shapes with ease
- A vegetable brush
- A compost can for the counter top (for you gardeners – even your flowers and shrubs will love it)
- Saucepan and skillet for the cooked vegan dishes

Just as I did, many of my vegan friends started with one sharp knife, a peeler, and a cutting board – and a burning desire to eat well, feel good and look great. That was it! If you don't have half of these appliances or tools right now, that's okay. Grab your knife and cutting board, and follow along.

Chapter 3: Go Cold Turkey or Ease into This?

I just hate to talk about calorie-counting, so I won't – except to say that if you go all-in as a vegan (particularly a raw vegan), you might not be eating enough calories every day for your body's energetic needs. A banana and 2 salads per day won't cut it! Water-rich raw vegetables have far fewer calories than you might guess. Even though you eat a lot of them, you might need more calories and feel, for a while, that you are "eating all the time".

Balance in All Things

Even if you go cooked, plan on consuming half of your calories as raw plant food (I am not including nuts here). If you are going raw vegan, plan on half of your daily calories coming from fruit. All vegans need to plan on half of your vegetables being green, preferably leafy but go with what you find. For most people, this all means they will be eating far more fruit in one day than they used to eat in one week, and far more greens! Don't worry – you will find your balance.

The most fat-rich (and calorie-rich as well) fruits and vegetables that you can eat are avocados, olives, nuts, and seeds like chia or flax. This said, don't overeat these foods on any given day. Or, if you happen to overeat any of them on one day, eliminate all of these foods on the following day. Balance in all things.

Smoothies

One great way to get balance – and enough calories – in your vegan way of eating is daily Smoothies. I am not adding smoothies to the recipe sections. This is because almost everyone has heard of smoothies, even though most people think of smoothies in terms of fruit only. Vegans, and particularly raw food Vegans, get a lot of their vegetables by drinking smoothies. If you can eat the vegetable raw, you can turn it into a smoothie. This has the advantage of getting more vegetables into your body than if you sat at a big salad bowl and ate the exact same amount of whole, raw vegetables or fruit.

First rule of the vegetable smoothie – don't expect it to be sweet! Expect it to taste like the vegetables in it. Second rule of the vegetable smoothie (all smoothies, in fact) – chew each mouthful before you swallow. That helps your whole digestive mechanism work on that fabulous nutrition.

Another aspect of balance as you become a vegan is **variety**. Maybe your mom and dad didn't buy any vegetables except carrots and tomatoes (and maybe an iceberg lettuce) when you were a kid. Just because you did not grow up seeing a wide range of fruit and vegetables on your table, doesn't mean you can't experiment now. The best way to explain this type of variety is to have a some of the following

fruit and vegetables on your plate every day:
- Fresh fruit
- Leafy greens
- 4 or more other colors and types of vegetables (not including white) with your greens at every meal
- Sprouts from seeds or pulses
- Sea vegetables

In spite of what I have just said about balance and variety, here is one last tip for successfully transitioning into your vegan life:

*Start, in all cases, by choosing foods that you **love to eat**!*

If you have never eaten seaweed for instance, and are not interested in such an adventure – skip it! Choose a more mouth-watering food.

Cold Turkey or Ease In?

There are really only two strategies for going vegan:

Jump in the deep end of this "vegan pool" right now. Toss or give away everything in your kitchen that is not Mother Nature's own fruit, vegetable, seed, or nut, and just have fun with creating tasty food every day.

The first strategy requires you to have some understanding of how much food you need to eat every day and what it looks like in your grocery cart – and your fridge and countertops. You will need to think about how much of your food is going to be cooked – and how you will make time to cook it – and how much of your food is going to be raw. You really, really need to plan ahead so that you always have plenty of food on hand – especially for when you travel for your job or get hungry when out shopping.

2. Slip down the "vegan pool" steps slowly from the shallow end, and wade slowly into the deep. You'll still empty

your cupboards, freezer, and fridge of all processed and refined and packaged foods that are on the No-Go list.

The second strategy allows you to start from where you are today in your eating habits. Do you eat meat? Do you eat it every day? One first step in this strategy might be to have a one-day-off / one-day-on approach to eating meat. On the days you do not eat meat, you will prepare a cooked vegan dish instead. If you eat a lot of dairy (milk products, cheeses, creams, yogurt), ween yourself off them in a similar way. No dairy on Monday, a little bit on Tuesday, and so on.

Another version of the second strategy is this. To remove all animal products and dairy from your diet, allow yourself one day per week to eat some meat, and a different day that week to have some dairy with your meal. Assign yet a different day in which to cook vegan if you are ultimately aiming for a raw-vegan-only life.

Your body might just sigh with relief when you do any of these. This plan might work better for you if you are still eating any of these eliminated foods, but not in great quantities.

Rush to Health

Some people have such an urgent need to eliminate their dangerous diagnoses and their symptoms and threats, that they go into an all-vegan (and maybe even all raw vegan) eating plan cold turkey. And they succeed! Other people need to slide gently into this change and get used to it gradually – but their health and wellness will still improve. I'll show you how to become a vegan either way.

Do a lot, and you get healthy faster, yes. Understand that going all-raw is the fastest way to recover your full health and skyrocket your energy levels. You could go all-raw overnight. Why not? However, if you are now on a heavy meat, dairy and processed foods pattern of eating, your body will be thrown into a bit of a tailspin. It is called "Detoxing" and it is not just for a body on drugs or booze! Your body will try to quickly eliminate the toxic fats, and all the overdoses of sugar and sodium you have been pouring into it for ... maybe your whole life. Give the body a break in this case, and go the cooked vegan route for several weeks or months first. Then, when you are out of the bathroom and more comfortable with that style of eating, you can transition to all-raw (if you wish).

Keep this in mind as you transition from your old way of eating to a Vegan Way:

Most vegans are going to thrive on some cooked plant foods, even if they are 95% raw vegans.

More on that next.

Chapter 4: Recipes – Cooked Transitioning

for Health

As I've stated several times, there are raw-food vegans who never take their food near an oven or stovetop, and other vegans who will cook some or all of their food (but who always start with food that is whole and raw fruit, vegetables, nuts, and seeds).

Let's look at some delicious all-vegan cooked recipes that are familiar even to meat eaters, and at how you can serve them up to increase the nutritional value of that entire meal.

Remember that you are going vegan for your health! Going vegan can and will provide you with very high levels of nutrition; your only job is to vary the types of raw fruit and vegetables that you eat so that you get the variety of nutritional elements as well. Going vegan is not about depriving yourself – as long as what you eat is as close to its natural, raw-plant form as possible.

The Vegan Kitchen

I have already listed in the previous chapter the appliances and utensils that will be useful to you in quickly preparing your vegan meals.

Here are the fresh, living herbs and plant spices that will help you create many a flavorful cooked vegan meal:

- Fresh herbs, however, you can find them (your garden, the produce section of the grocer's). These include fresh basil, rosemary, thyme, sage. I would include all types of parsley here, such as Italian, frizzy and cilantro.
- Spicy stuff – hot chili peppers of any "temperature" that you feel like experimenting with.
- Spices without heat, such as nutmeg, cinnamon, and natural vanilla bean...

NOTE: To encourage yourself to <u>stop salting</u> your food, have **fresh** lemons for lemon juice in the house at all times. Yes, it is a different flavor from salt, I get that. Yes, it will help you get away from the need to salt all your food. Just try it!

Here is where to start shopping for this luscious, delicious raw food:

- Asian markets
- Farmer's markets
- Buy from a food co-op (and volunteer there for even cheaper food)
- Buy organic as often as you have access to it and can afford it
- Grow your own food – from organic seeds

Recipes

Citrus Zing Salad Dressing

- Juice of two lemons
- Juice of any additional citrus fruit, like grapefruit, orange, tangerine, etc.
- 1/4 – 1/2 teaspoon cayenne pepper or crushed black peppers

This is a no-salt, no deprivation basic salad dressing. You can make this one of two ways.

First way: use a citrus juicer and use only the juice of the fruit; stir in the pepper.

Second way: use a blender; peel the fruit; blend till liquid, seeds and all. If you blend it, toss in the pepper at the same time.

Store in the fridge in a glass jar or Tupperware. Serving this on any raw vegetable salad – especially a salad with some sharp vegetables like radishes or onion – creates a zingy flavor on your tongue.

Variation

If you have a blender, add a **half a cup of cashew nuts** to the above recipe.

NOTE: Whenever you eat nuts, make sure you soak them for 2-4 hours in plain room-temperature water before consuming them. This simply makes them more digestible to our human tummies. Drain the water off (I have never heard that the water retains any nutritional value).

Also, try adding this version to any mostly-vegetable salad with whole pieces of citrus fruit in it. We forget that we can mix fruit and vegetables for a tasty treat.

Tomato-Herb Dressing

Some of my friends also call this a "fresh salsa."

- Green parsley of your choice, a small bunch – fine chopped
- Fresh tomatoes, 2 cups when rough chopped
- 2-3 green onions – fine chopped
- One garlic clove – crushed and fine chopped

Just stir all the chopped ingredients together in a big bowl, and give the whole thing a couple hours in the fridge or 30 minutes on the countertop so that the flavors blend.

All you really need to make this dressing is a sharp knife, but if you are good with the chopping function of a food processor, you can certainly use one to go faster. I do not purée these ingredients, but just chop them finely. The raw tomato makes enough juice for it to become a "salad dressing".

Variation

Could you eat this straight out of the blender as a chopped salad in its own right? Absolutely!

Don't forget you can also pour it on your raw all-veg or fruit plus veg salads. Toss it well, let it sit for 15 minutes and then dive in for a tasty meal.

Pour this dressing onto some fresh-cooked quinoa (see below) and chow down. Yummy!

Main Courses

Quinoa and Pulses

Say KEEN-wah. I have never seen quinoa for sale in the United States that is not organic. Pulses are the various types of lentils – pink, golden, brown – garbanzo beans, other dried beans, and dried peas. In the United States, most of these are traditionally grown (not guaranteed to be organic).

There is no need to soak quinoa. Cook it like you do rice - 1 cup of dry quinoa to 2 cups of water, over a simmering heat. You will know the quinoa is done when it smells nutty and the grains easily crush when you pitch them with your fingers. It should not be mushy!

Variation:

I often make huge pots of broth-rich vegetable soup. Cook your dry quinoa in this nutritious broth instead of filtered water! Yummy.

You should soak all your pulses, from 2-4 hours, drain them, and simmer them on a medium heat in fresh water. Like nuts, soaking pulses makes them more digestible for our human tummies. While the water for the beans or pulses is heating up, rough-chop the following vegetables and throw them in the pot. The quantities are per person:

- 2 large carrots
- 1/2 onion
- 3 cloves of garlic, crushed
- 1 branch fresh thyme, one bay leaf, 1 teaspoon or one branch of rosemary
- A pinch or two of cayenne pepper

The beans are done when you blow on one and the skin curls back – or when the bean itself is soft on the tongue.

Serve up a big scoop of quinoa next to a big scoop of seasoned pulses. There is no added salt, fat or oil, or artificial anything! Guilt-free eating!

While you're waiting for the quinoa to finish cooking, serve up a raw veg salad so that you get the best of both raw and cooked vegan worlds.

Variation – Breakfast

One of my cooked vegan friends loves warm or cold quinoa for breakfast! She tends to pile fresh berries on top of a bowl of this grain or to eat a huge bowl of raw fresh fruit on the side. That's breakfast. Try it – it is filling, satisfying, protein-rich. It is sweet but sugar-free. And like the next variation, it sticks to your ribs all morning.

A variation on pulses is a breakfast favorite of the vegan crowd. I prefer this breakfast with lentils and carrots only. If you have also stewed some tomatoes and fresh thyme into the dish, it doesn't matter — heat up a big bowl of this soup on a cold winter morning, and you have a hearty, satisfying substitute for sugary, buttery oatmeal with milk.

Mashups and Steamers

This is not so much a recipe but some preparation guidelines for getting more variety out of the "same old" vegetables.

One preparation is what I call **mashups**. It is inspired by traditional mashed potatoes but uses other nontraditional vegetables. Here is an example:

- 4 leaves of frizzy kale, with stems if not too thick
- 2 heads of broccoli, florets and stems

Boil water in a saucepan. You are not cooking the kale and broccoli, but blanching them. This means you are dipping the broccoli into the boiling water until it turns bright green. You are dipping the frizzy kale into the boiling water until it likewise turns a brighter green and softens a very tiny bit.

Now, chop the broccoli and kale and put it in your blender. Lightly pulse it — be careful not to liquefy it! You want a chunk or two to remain. Scoop it out onto a plate as your hot side vegetable.

That's one type of mashup and a good way to get lots of greens if you're not otherwise inclined to eat broccoli or kale!

Take this same approach with zucchini. You can also do it with cauliflower or any color of cabbage. Heat it up in boiling water, blanch it, and toss it in the blender. That's it.

Steamers start with vegetables that you simply prefer to eat in their cooked form — carrots, potatoes, onions, cabbage, cauliflower, mustard greens and so on.

To make steamers, you need a big pot or rice cooker and a steamer tray that fits in the bottom of the pot. You can buy these at any grocery store (it is usually one size fits all pots). The point is, you are not boiling these vegetables in lots of water. It is the steam that is cooking your vegetables. You will discover, if you don't already know this, that steaming keeps the flavors in the vegetables much better than boiling ever could!

Peel and cut your vegetables into bite-size pieces. Put an inch of water in the bottom of the pot and put the steamer tray on top of that. Remember which vegetables take longest to cook and put those in the steamer tray first. This would include potatoes and carrots and thick slices of cabbage. Layer the other vegetables on top of these.

Toss in some herbs — laurel, mint, rosemary...

Since you have cut vegetables into bite-size pieces, keep an eye on cooking progress — it will go fast once the water boils. When the vegetables are soft to your liking, pull the tray up and out of the pot. Eat the vegetables with any raw salad dressing you like!

Stewed Red Sauce

Contrary to all the tomato sauces in cans, this one is chock-full of garden-fresh raw vegetables – and totally free of added salt, sugars or sweeteners, and fat. With this sauce, you truly get your daily supply of many other vegetables.

- 2 pounds ripe red tomatoes, any variety
- 1 pound carrots, grated or fine sliced in food processor
- 1/2 cabbage, fine sliced
- 1-2 onions, fine sliced
- Fresh (not dried) Italian herbs of your choice, such as thyme, rosemary, basil, any type of parsley
- 2-5 cloves of garlic – optional
- fresh chili pepper, any type – optional (for those of you who like spice)

I say to slice or grate all of these ingredients because you are now going to layer them in a crockpot or slow cooker. Set the dial on low and walk away for 6 to 8 hours. If you need to do this on the stovetop in a cooking pot, be sure to put juicy tomatoes on the bottom of the pot first. Set the flame or heat on the lowest possible temperature, cover the pot and check on it every two hours or so.

This is, of course, a cooked vegan dish. It can be eaten on its own hot or cold. I just like to wrap it in a big romaine or chard leaf and munch away.

Variations:

Blend it up smooth or keep it chunky.
If you want to venture into raw-vegan territory, and have purchased a spiralizer – Spiralize two or three (raw, of course!) zucchini or summer squash. Pour the sauce, hot or cold, over the raw zucchini

that you have turned into "spaghetti, fettuccine or wide noodle slices" with your spiralizer. Mix well, and dive in with a fork and knife.

Spoon some of this tomato-rich sauce over your power pate (raw recipe chapter) or into your cooked lentil stew.

Vegan Lasagna

You can literally make this with any sliceable vegetables that you have in the refrigerator. I will show you how to do this with winter vegetables.

- 1 onion, any color
- 1/2 cabbage, any color
- Several leaves of kale, any type (no stems)
- 3 potatoes
- 2-3 yams or sweet potatoes
- Herbs of any type you enjoy – basil, thyme, rosemary – about 2 tablespoons altogether
- Cayenne or black pepper to taste – or chili peppers – your choice

- A dash of powdered cinnamon (I add this to the tomato sauce first)
- 1-2 cups of your homemade tomato sauce
- Crushed garlic – optional

Start with whole vegetables for this recipe. Peel the onion and potatoes. Slice all the vegetables into quarter inch slices. Layer them in an oven dish any way you like, covering each layer with tomato sauce and some herbs and pepper (and garlic, optional).

I like to bake this at 200° for several hours because everything just melts into each other – all the while preserving the individual flavors of vegetables. You can bake it at 350° for an hour if you like vegetables crunchy. Add 30 minutes if you prefer them softer.

Yes, it is a cooked dish. You can serve it to non-vegan friends without blushing. You can eat it yourself without feeling any guilt. There is no cheese. There is no oil. There is no salt. There is no sugar in your homemade tomato sauce. A healthy, tasty winner!

Chapter 5: Recipes – Raw, Living, Energizing and Delicious

It is always a good idea as a vegan to consume 50% of your daily foods in raw form. You're going for better, improved health and the nutrition is in the raw stuff! (Reminder: zero natural nutrition remains in factory-processed foods, no matter what type of "nutritional supplements" they add or what type of packaging it ends up in).

As an all-vegan, all-raw individual, you can eat most pulses and many dried beans by sprouting them. Add them to your sprouted seeds (radish, alfalfa and so on), and you have powerful nutrition.

You can whizz up your own fresh salad dressings in the blender from raw vegetables and fruits – and why not a few nuts or seeds? Even your dips and salad dressings are made, as you will see, from raw, whole, real foods. That means that you could easily eat any of these salad dressings with a spoon as a meal! I'm not sure you would like to do that when your factory-processed, store-bought salad dressing comes out of a bottle filled with oil, sodium, and sugar!

Here are some delicious ways to eat your meals in raw forms. As a raw-food vegan, remember that everything that you eat is "just Mother Nature's own food".

Contrary to others, a raw-food vegan will rarely, if ever, use bottled oils, or any bottled, canned or packaged condiment or ingredient in his food. These recipes take that preference into account.

The Vegan Kitchen

The same living, raw herbs and spices used by a cooked-food vegan are the same — except that you will find yourself consuming more of them!

Recipes

Salad Dressings

Eating raw becomes a pleasure of a higher order when you start to invent salad dressings from real, living, edible foods. I cannot tell you the number of times I have sat with a bowl of "salad dressing" and polished it off... Without the salad! All of these recipes are real food. Whether you become an all-raw or a cooked vegan, add these living salad dressings to your routine.

Cherry Tomato Beet Top Dressing

- 2 cups or about a pound and a half tomatoes
- Handful beet or mustard greens, Swiss chard leaves (no hard stems) – rough chopped
- 4 celery stalks – rough chopped
- 1 tablespoon fresh lemon juice
- 1/4 cup packed fresh cilantro – stems are okay

Blend all ingredients at once on the highest speed until smooth. Use immediately, or you can refrigerate for a day or two.

Yellow Bell Pepper Mango Dressing

- 2 large mangoes – peeled, pitted, cut into chunks
- 1 yellow bell pepper – rough chopped
- 3 tablespoons raw sesame seeds – or cashews, crushed
- 1 stem fresh rosemary leaves

Blend all ingredients at once on the highest speed until smooth. Use immediately, or you can refrigerate it for a day or two.

I have replaced the mangoes with papayas with tasty success, too.

Raw Veg with Amazing Dips

Just because you are an all-raw vegan (or simply having an all-raw vegan day today only), some of your friends will think that everything you eat is a "Salad". Don't let them tease you too much, but do let them see the big smile on your face when you dip some raw veg into these outrageously delicious all-food dips. No added fats, salt, sugar – and nothing artificial! Pure, nutritious food…that just tastes sinful.

BLENDING TIP:

If at the beginning of your vegan journey your only appliance is a blender, here is a way to get more action from your blender with non-juicy vegetables and fruit.

For hard vegetables like broccoli, cauliflower, onions, carrots (you get the idea), first chop them into golf-ball sized chunks; put them in the blender. Fill the blender with water - really just to cover the vegetables in the blender jar. Start the blender on low, and you will see how the chunks swirl down to the blades through the whirlpool action of the water. It won't take long! Use a low speed! Empty the contents of the blender into a strainer. Now you have rice-sized bits of hard vegetables that can be blended much more easily with nuts, other water-logged vegetables or flavored liquids.

Cashew Cheese

- Head of cauliflower – thick stem removed
- 1 c cashews – soaked and drained
- 1-2 cloves garlic – crushed
- 1/4 - 1/3 onion

Water-blend the cauliflower to a rice size and drain the water; return it to the blender with other ingredients. Blend all ingredients together into a creamy "cheesy" dip. Don't forget the garlic – it is the "secret" to this dip!

No-Bean Bean Dip

- 1 large or 2 medium zucchini – cut in chunks
- 1 cup raw sesame or sunflower seeds
- 1/2 cup fresh lemon juice – about two lemons
- 1 garlic clove – crushed

Blend all ingredients at once on high speed until smooth. Eat immediately, or refrigerate for up to 2 days. This tastes a little like garbanzo bean hummus.

I have replaced the seeds with 3-4 tablespoons tahini (less, since it is more concentrated). Still great!

NOTE: How to sprout seeds

Any of the beans/seeds I have talked about sprout fairly quickly in three days maximum. Whichever type you choose, soak them for 4 to 6 hours in room temperature water first. I like to change the water every hour. Then drain off the water by pouring the beans into a colander (plastic or metal is fine). Cover the colander with a wet paper towel or dishrag and set the colander over a bowl to capture any dripping moisture. Once or twice a day, take the towel off and rinse the beans under running water. Just cover them up again and watch the little tails (sprouts) form. When the tails are an eighth to a quarter inch long, you are ready to just eat the sprouts, or use them in any recipe like the Power Pate recipe below.

This is the basic process I use for all of my sprouting. Since different beans sprout over different periods, I tend to keep them separate from each other. The process is exactly the same for quinoa, chickpeas and so on. My all-time favorite for sprouting are mung and lentils. Both are quickly sprouted, and I just like the way they taste! For a recipe like Power Pate, they are both easily crushed into pate as well.

Power Pate

Perhaps years and years ago you went to one of the Western world's first vegan restaurants. If so, you probably saw a mountain of brown goo, that was actually lentils which had simply been puréed. Here is a much more nutritious (since raw) and appetizing version, which is a delicious dish for the all-raw vegan and the cooked vegan alike.

For best success and fastest results, you will need a food processor rather than a blender. I give you here the proportions – you can cut everything in half or double everything depending on who you are preparing the dish for.

- 4 – 6 cups sprouted sunflower seeds, lentils or mung beans
- 2 bell peppers (any color but green), rough chopped
- 2 to 4 cloves crushed garlic
- 2 to 3 carrots, grated

- 2 to 3 thick slices of onion – any type you like
- One branch celery with leaves, rough chopped
- A huge bunch of any type of parsley (Italian, frizzy or cilantro)
- Juice of half a lemon
- 1/2 to 1 teaspoon crushed black pepper or cayenne pepper to taste

Toss all the water-logged vegetables you have rough-chopped in the bottom of the blender first. Give them a quick blend. Now add the sprouts. The liquid from the water-rich veg will help you pull in and purée the sprouts next. You want, however, to achieve a fairly dry, homogeneous mixture. It is the raw vegetarian equivalent of a meat pate, please recall!

Taste your raw mixture and adjust the seasoning. I find I typically like more parsley or more of the bitter taste of celery leaves. You may find that you prefer the added kick of more cayenne pepper.

This is a basic recipe, as most of these in this book are! Play with it.

3 Ways to Enjoy Pate

Wraps

For lunch or dinner, scoop some of this powerfully nutritious, filling pate onto a whole leaf of romaine lettuce, or a leaf of chard — fold the leafy green around the pate and munch. It is a raw-vegan burrito or bread-free sandwich.

Dips

Scoop some pate into a wide slice of bell pepper, or onto a zucchini or celery stick. The pate is a dip for veggie sticks.

Sushi

Spread this pate on a raw Nori sheet (raw seaweed) with other thin sliced or grated raw vegetables. Roll it up, slice it up and munch. You have delicious sushi.

Basic Fruit Pudding

Go back to what I said about Chia seeds and flax seeds. A shared characteristic of these two seeds is that they thicken foods that contain water. Pour water on the seeds, and they thicken all on their own, too. That makes them perfect for creating a raw-vegan pudding! Here is a basic fruit pudding recipe using bananas. Just swap out the quantity of bananas with any other fruit you like, including dried fruits such as dates, raisins or apricots. In winter, I like to mix fresh fruit like bananas with dried fruit for an extra rich and satisfying pudding. If you want to add dried fruit to your pudding, first soak them for 15 minutes in warm water to soften them up.

2 tablespoons whole or ground Chia seeds, or ground flax seeds
2 cups fresh bananas
1/4 cup filtered water (or other fruit juice that you have made yourself from a juicer)
a dash of ground cinnamon (optional)

Soak the seeds in the filtered water for 10 minutes. You will notice that the water thickens. Pour the seeds and water into the blender along with your choice of fruit. Blend thoroughly (with cinnamon, if you use it), and let it sit for 20 minutes. Blend again and then pour into a refrigerator container. Let it chill for a couple of hours, then dive in.

Another guilt free treat, since there is no added sweetener – it is all just Mother Nature's real food.

I have made this pudding with bananas, berries, dried fruit only, berries plus avocado, and apples. Experiment!

Conclusion
A Weird New Kitchen

Of course, your routine-oriented brain will try to convince you that you are deprived as you persist on eating cooked vegan or raw vegan ways because you no longer swing into the fast-food carryout lane for a quick meal. With the wealth of raw fruit and vegetables in our supermarkets nowadays and your own ability to create a food garden (even on your balcony – and it is a huge urban trend), there is no excuse for caving into that routine-oriented brain of yours.

You won't be eating any meat or other animal products. You will probably have thrown out or given away your formerly-favorite processed condiments and snacks, breakfast foods and packets of just-add-water cookables. Your freezer has no store-bought containers in it anymore. Your fridge looks "weird", because all that is in it now is fresh (and quickly perishable) fruit and vegetables. All that is in your cupboard are sproutable beans, nuts, and seeds!

Research on Real Food

I have waited until the end of the book to prove to you with scientific evidence that you can do this, you can regain and retain your health, you can reduce or eliminate your diagnoses and the related symptoms they present, you can and will lose weight healthfully – and in the process, you will never feel deprived.

Our nutritional mistreatment of our bodies is not an American phenomenon only. For this reason, I am listing for you studies that looked at mainland Chinese, American, European and New Zealand populations.

Part 2

Introduction

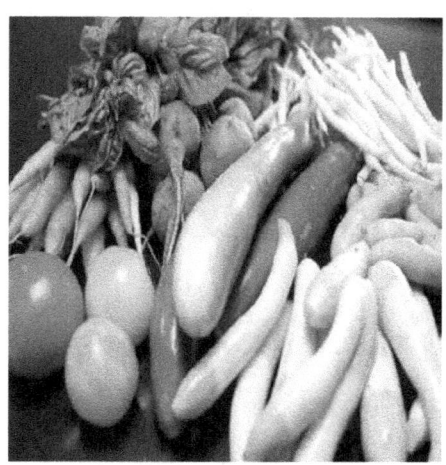

With many people switching over to the vegan lifestyle, it is not hard to see why it is becoming one of the most popular lifestyles to follow today. The main reason why many people are turning to the vegan lifestyle is because of the vast benefits associated with it. If this is the reason you are interested in switching to the vegan lifestyle and only consuming vegan friendly foods, then this is certainly the book for you.

Inside of this book you will learn not only how to make some of the most delicious vegan recipes you will ever find, but you will also discover a few vegan friendly dishes that will help you to make healthy food conscious decision to enjoying the healthiest foods possible.

So, without further ado, let's get right to cooking!

Delicious Vegan Recipes

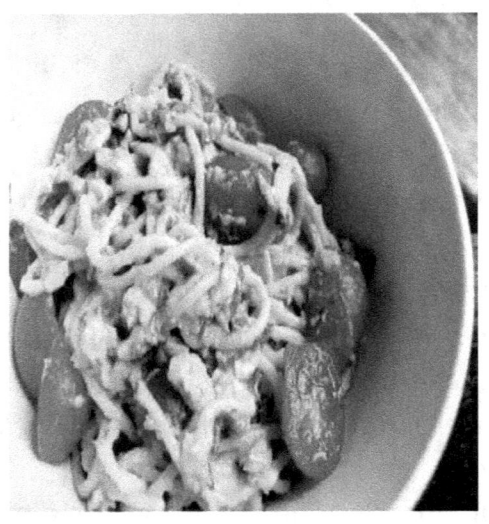

Sweet Tasting Carrot Risotto

Here is a sweet and filling vegan style

breakfast dish that I know you are going to love. Simple to make and packed full of delicious taste, this is one dish that you are going to want to make over and over again.

Makes: 4 Servings

Total Prep Time: 35 Minutes

Ingredients:

- ¼ Cup + 1 Tbsp. of Olive Oil, Extra Virgin Variety
- 1 Cup of Onion, White in Color and Finely Diced
- 1 Tbsp. of Garlic, Minced
- 2 Cups of Rice, Arborio Variety
- 1/3 Cup of Wine, White in Color
- 1 Tbsp. of Lemon Juice, Fresh
- 1 ½ Quarts of Carrot Stock, Fresh and Homemade Preferable
- 1 Cup of Carrot Juice, Fresh
- ¼ Cup of Carrots, Finely Diced
- Dash of Salt, For Taste
- 1 Tbsp. of Thyme, Fresh

Directions:

1. Use a large sized skillet and heat up at least ¼ cup of your oil over medium heat. Once your oil is hot enough add in your onions and cook them until they are translucent.

2. Then add in your garlic and cook for an additional minute or until fragrant.

3. Next add in your rice and stir to thoroughly coat. Continue to cook until translucent.

4. Add in your wine and stir again to incorporate. Cook until your liquid has fully evaporated. Then add in your lemon juice and continue to cook until the liquid has fully evaporated.

5. Next slowly add in your carrot stock. Stir again to incorporate before adding in your finely diced carrots. Continue to cook for another 10 minutes.

6. Add in your remaining oil and season with a dash of salt for taste.

7. Remove from heat and serve with a garnish of thyme. Enjoy while still piping hot.

Savory Blueberry Scones

If you are a huge fan of the scones that are often served up at your local Starbucks, then I know you are going to love this recipe. Packed full of fresh blueberries and sweet to taste, I know you are going to want to enjoy these scones with your morning coffee.

Makes: 6 to 7 Servings
Total Prep Time: 30 Minutes
Ingredients:
- 1 ¾ Cups of Flour, All Purpose Variety
- ¾ Cup of Oats, Quick Cooking Variety
- ½ tsp. of Baker's Style Baking Soda
- 2 tsp. of Baker's Style Baking Powder
- Dash of Salt, For Taste
- ¾ Cup of Sugar, White in Color
- ½ Cup of Margarine, Soft
- 2 Tbsp. of Lemon Juice, Fresh
- ½ Cup of Milk, Soy Variety
- 1 Cup of Blueberries, Fresh

Directions:

1. First preheat your oven to 400 degrees. While your oven is heating up grease a large sized cookie sheet with a generous amount of cooking spray.

2. Then use a large sized bowl and add in your flour, oats, baker's style baking soda, baker's style baking powder and dash of salt. Stir thoroughly to combine.

3. Add in your sugar, butter, fresh lemon juice and soy milk. Stir again to incorporate.

4. Gently fold in your blueberries, making sure not to overmix.

5. Drop your dough by the spoonful onto your greased cookie sheet.

6. Place into your oven to bake for the next 10 to 15 minutes or until your scones are lightly brown on top.

7. Remove and allow to cool slightly before serving.

Streusel Topped Coffee Cake

If you are looking for a vegan style recipe that the entire family can enjoy, then this is the perfect dish for you to enjoy. Feel free to serve this dish with your favorite icing to make the tastiest results.

Makes: 12 Servings

Total Prep Time: 40 Minutes

Ingredients:
- 1 Cup of Milk, Soy Variety
- 1 Tbsp. of Vinegar, White in Color and Distilled
- 1/3 Cup of Tofu, Soft
- 2 ¼ Cups of Flour, All Purpose Variety
- 1 ¼ Cups of Brown Sugar, Light and packed
- 3 tsp. of Cinnamon, Evenly Divided
- 1 ½ tsp. of Ginger, Ground Variety
- ½ tsp. of Salt, For Taste
- ¾ Cup of Oil, Vegetable Variety
- ¾ Cup of Walnuts, Finely Chopped

- 1 tsp. of Baker's Style Baking Powder
- 1 tsp. of Baker's Style Baking Soda

Directions:

1. First preheat your oven to 350 degrees. While your oven is heating up grease a large sized baking dish and set aside for later use.

2. Then add your milk, vinegar and tofu into a blender. Blend on the highest setting until smooth in consistency.

3. Then use a large sized bowl and add in your flour, light brown sugar, cinnamon, ginger, dash of salt and oil. Stir thoroughly to mix.

4. Transfer at least 1 ¼ cups of this mixture into a small sized bowl. Add your remaining cinnamon and walnuts to this mixture. Stir thoroughly to incorporate.

5. Add your baker's style baking powder, baker's style baking soda and tofu mixture into your remaining flour mixture. Stir until your mixture is smooth in consistency.

6. Pour your batter into your baking dish and pour your nut mixture over the top.

7. Place into your oven to bake for the next 30 to 35 minutes or until completely cooked through.

8. Remove from oven and allow to cool slightly before serving. Enjoy.

Orange Style French Toast

While I know this may not seem like a wholly satisfying dish, I know you won't be able to get enough of it. For the tastiest results I highly recommend garnishing with a generous amount of powdered sugar before serving.

Makes: 3 Servings

Total Prep Time: 15 Minutes

Ingredients:

- 1, 6 Inch Slices of French Bread
- ¼ Cup of Cream Cheese, Nondairy Variety
- ½ tsp. of Orange Peel, Finely Shredded
- 1 ½ tsp. of Orange Juice, Fresh
- 5 Tbsp. of Sugar, White in Color

- ½ Cup of Milk, Soy Variety
- 3 Tbsp. of Flour, Unbleached Variety
- 1 tsp. of Vanilla, Pure
- Some Vegan Friendly Margarine, For Cooking
- Dash of Confectioner's Sugar, For Garnish
- Some Strawberries, Fresh and for Garnish

Directions:

1. The first thing that you will want to do is cut a small pocket horizontally into each slice of your bread. Make sure that you do not cut all the way through your bread. Set aside for later use.

2. Then use a small sized bowl and add in your cream cheese, orange peel, fresh orange juice and white sugar. Stir thoroughly to combine and spoon this mixture into the pockets of your bread slices.

3. Next use a shallow bowl and add in your milk, flour and vanilla. Use an electric

mixer and blend on the highest setting until smooth in consistency.

4. Add your bread slices into your soy milk mixture and allow to soak for the next 5 seconds on one side before turning over. Allow to soak for another 5 seconds.

5. Melt your vegan margarine in a large sized griddle placed over medium heat. Once it is hot enough add your bread slices and cook for at least 3 to 4 minutes on each side or until golden brown in color.

6. Remove and serve with a sprinkling of your confectioner's sugar. Garnish with your fresh strawberries and serve right away.

Vegan Style Banana Bread

If you are a huge fan of traditional banana bread, then this is one dish that you are going to fall in love with. Easy to make and completely filling, this is one breakfast dish you are going to want to make all of the time.

Makes: 6 to 8 Servings

Total Prep Time: 1 Hour and 10 Minutes

Ingredients:

- 1 Tbsp. of Flaxseed, Ground Variety + 3 Tbsp. of Water
- 3 to 4 Bananas, Ripe and Mashed
- 1/6 Cup of Oil, Canola Variety
- 1/6 Cup of Applesauce, Unsweetened Variety
- ½ Cup of Agave Nectar
- 1 tsp. of Vanilla, Pure
- 1 tsp. of Baker's Style Baking Soda
- 1 ½ Cups of Flour, Whole Wheat Variety
- ¼ tsp. of Salt, For Taste
- ¾ Cup of Walnuts, Cut into Small Sized Pieces and Optional
- ½ Cup of Chocolate Chips, Optional

Directions:

1. Use a small sized bowl and add in your flaxseed with your water. Stir well to combine and cover with some plastic wrap. Place into your fridge to chill for at

least one hour. After this time remove and stir.

2. Then preheat your oven to 325 degrees.

3. Next use a large sized bowl and add in your mashed bananas, oil, unsweetened applesauce, nectar and pure vanilla. Add in your flaxseed mixture and stir well to combine.

4. Add in your flour, baker's style baking soda and salt. Stir well until evenly combined.

5. Grease a large sized bread pan with a generous amount of cooking spray. Pour your mixture into your greased bread pan.

6. Place into your oven to bake for the next 45 to 55 minutes or until your bread is completely baked through.

7. Remove and allow to cool slightly before slicing.

Matzo Meal Pancakes

If you are a huge fan of pancakes, then this

is one Vegan recipe I know you are going to be craving more. Serve these pancakes with your favorite syrup for the tastiest results.

Makes: 12 Servings

Total Prep Time: 10 Minutes

Ingredients:

- 1 ½ Cups of Matzo Meal
- ¼ Cup of Sugar, White in Color
- 4 tsp. of Baker's Style Baking Powder
- 3 Cups of Water, Warm
- ½ Cups of Apples, Minced
- 1 tsp. of Cinnamon, Ground
- Some Oil, For Frying

Directions:

1. Use a large sized bowl and add in all of your ingredients except for your oil. Stir well to combine.

2. Next heat up your oil in a large sized frying pan. Once the oil is hot enough add in spoonfuls of your batter to your pan and flatten with a spoon.

3. Cook your pancakes until brown in color. This should take at least 2 minutes.

4. After this time flip and continue to cook on the other side for another 2 minutes.

5. Remove and repeat until all of your batter has been used.

6. Serve with your favorite syrup and enjoy.

Sticky Cinnamon Buns

Have a few picky eaters in your household? Then this is the perfect dish for you to make. It is so easy to make that even your children are going to want to help out in the kitchen.

Makes: 12 Servings

Total Prep Time: 25 Minutes

Ingredients:

- 1 1/3 Cups of Sugar, Granulated Variety
- 3 Tbsp. of Cinnamon, Ground
- 3 Cans of Biscuits, Refrigerated Variety

- ½ Cup of Margarine, Nondairy Variety and Fully Melted
- 1 Cup of Confectioner's Sugar
- 2 to 3 tsp. of Milk, Soy Variety

Directions:

1. First preheat your oven to 350 degrees. While your oven is heating up oil a large sized cupcake pan with a generous amount of oil and set aside for later use.

2. Then mix together your sugar and cinnamon in a small sized container.

3. Cut each of your biscuits into four equal sized pieces. Place your biscuit pieces into your container and shake thoroughly to coat. Transfer your biscuit pieces into your greased cupcake pan.

4. Use a medium sized bowl and combine your remaining ingredients into your sugar and cinnamon mixture. Stir thoroughly to combine and pour at least a spoonful into each muffin tin.

5. Place into your oven to bake for the next 10 minutes or until slightly brown in color.

6. After this time remove from your oven and allow to cool slightly before transferring to a plate.

7. Use a small sized bowl and mix your confectioner's sugar with some soy milk, stirring well to form a glaze. Drizzle your glaze over your buns.

8. Serve immediately and enjoy.

Vegan Style Pumpkin Spiced Pancakes

Here is yet another pancake recipe I know you are going to fall in love with. It is the perfect pancake recipe to make whenever pumpkin comes into season.

Makes: 12 Servings

Total Prep Time: 18 Minutes

Ingredients:

- 1 ½ Cups of Milk, Vanilla and Almond Variety
- 2 Tbsp. of Vinegar
- 1 Cup of Pumpkin, Puree Variety
- 2 Tbsp. of Margarine, Vegan Variety and Fully Melted

- 2 Tbsp. of Maple Syrup
- 1 tsp. of Vanilla, Pure
- 2 Tbsp. of Oil, Vegetable Variety
- 3 Tbsp. of Brown Sugar, Light and Packed
- 2 Cups of Flour, Whole Wheat Variety
- 1 tsp. of Baker's Style Baking Soda
- 2 tsp. of Baker's Style Baking Powder
- ½ tsp. of Salt, For Taste
- 2 ¼ tsp. of Pumpkin Pie Spice

Directions:

1. The first thing that you will want to do is use a large sized bowl and add in your almond milk, pumpkin, margarine, maple syrup, pure vanilla, vinegar and oil. Stir thoroughly to combine and set aside for later use.

2. Using a separate bowl add in your brown sugar, flour, baker's style baking soda, baker's style baking powder, dash of salt and pumpkin pie spice. Stir thoroughly to combine.

3. Add this mixture to your wet mixture and stir again to incorporate. Allow to sit for the next 5 to 10 minutes.

4. Next spray a large sized skillet with a generous amount of cooking spray. Set over medium heat and once it is hot enough add in at least ¼ cup of your batter. Cook until bubbles begin to form on the surface. Flip and continue to cook for an additional 3 to 5 minutes.

5. Repeat until all of your batter has been used.

6. Serve your pancakes with your favorite maple syrup and a dash of pumpkin spice. Enjoy.

Vegan Style Chicken Alfredo Lasagna Rolls

If you are a huge fan of chicken alfredo, then this is the perfect dish for you. This absolutely delicious meal makes enough that your entire family will fall in love with.

Makes: 6 Servings

Total Prep Time: 35 Minutes

Ingredients:

- 1 pack of Tofu, Extra Firm Variety and Drained
- 8 Ounces of Spinach, Fresh and Finely Chopped
- 1 tsp. of Garlic, Minced
- 2 tsp. of Lemon Juice, Fresh
- ½ Cup of Yeast, Nutritional Variety
- Dash of Salt and Pepper, For Taste
- 1 Cup of Cashews, soaked in Water and Drained
- ¼ Cup of Milk, Nondairy Variety
- 1 Package of Lasagna Noodles, Fully Cooked and Drained
- 1 Package of Chicken Strips, Vegan Style
- Some Parsley, Fresh and Roughly Chopped

Directions:

1. The first thing that you will want to do is preheat your oven to 350 degrees.

2. While your oven is heating up add your tofu, fresh spinach, garlic, fresh lemon juice, yeast, dash of salt and dash of pepper into a large sized bowl. Mix this

mixture using your hands and stir well until crumbled. Set aside for later use.

3. Add in your cashews, milk garlic, fresh lemon juice, salt, pepper, and yeast unto a blender. Blend on the highest setting until smooth in consistency. Add more milk for your mixture to reach its desired consistency.

4. Spread some of your tofu mixture onto your lasagna noodles followed by three pieces of your vegan chicken. Roll your noodles and place into a large sized baking dish. Repeat until your dish is filled with rolls.

5. Pour your freshly made sauce over the top.

6. Place into your oven to bake for the next 20 to 25 minutes or until piping hot.

7. Remove and allow to cool slightly. Top off with your freshly parsley and serve whenever you are ready. Enjoy.

Vegan Style Cheese Stuffed Burger

This is a great tasting vegan style burger recipe to make if you love the taste of burgers in general. Feel free to top this burger off with your choice of toppings for the tastiest results.

Makes: 1 Serving

Total Prep Time: 18 Minutes

Ingredients:
- 2 Burger Patties, Vegan Style
- 2 Ounces of Vegan Style Cheese
- 1 Hamburger Bun
- Toppings of Your Choice

Directions:

1. Make a small indentation in the center of your burger patties and place your vegan cheese into it.

2. Top off with your second burger patty.

3. Place onto a preheat grill set over medium heat and cook for at least 8 minutes before flipping. Continue to cook for an additional 8 minutes on the other side or until your cheese is fully melted.

4. Remove and serve on your favorite burger bun. Top off with your favorite toppings and enjoy right away.

Easy Vegan Mac and Cheese

Do you love the savory taste of mac and cheese? Then this is the perfect dish for you to make. Smothered in delicious Vegan style cheese and topped off with some cashews, I know you won't be able to get enough of it.

Makes: 6 Servings

Total Prep Time: 20 Minutes

Ingredients:

- 1 Clove of Garlic
- 1 tsp. of Turmeric
- ½ tsp. of Salt, For Taste
- ¼ Cup of Yeast, Nutritional Variety
- 1 Cup of Cashews, Soaked and Drained
- ¼ Cup of Water, Warm
- 1, 8 Ounce Pack of Pasta, Cooked and Drained

Directions:

1. Place your garlic, salt, yeast, nuts, water and turmeric into a blender.
2. Blend on the highest setting until smooth in consistency.
3. Pour this mixture over your cooked and hot pasta, tossing well to combine.
4. Heat thoroughly before serving.

Healthy Avocado Pesto Pasta

If you are a huge fan of Avocado and Pesto, then this is one dish that I know you are definitely going to want to try for yourself. It is easy to make and packed full of a delicious flavor that you won't be able to resist.

Makes: 3 Servings

Total Prep Time: 12 Minutes

Ingredients:

- 1 Pound Of Linguine, Uncooked Variety

- 1 Bunch of Basil, Fresh and Some for Garnish
- ½ Cup of Nuts, Pine Variety
- 2 Avocados, Pitted and Peeled
- 2 Tbsp. of Lemon Juice, Fresh
- 3 Cloves of Garlic, Minced
- ½ Cup of Olive Oil, Extra Virgin Variety
- Dash of Sea Salt, For Taste
- Dash of Black Pepper, For Taste
- 1 Cup of Tomatoes, Cherry Variety

Directions:

1. The first thing that you will want to do is bring a large sized pot of water to a boil. Add in a touch of salt and add in your linguine. Cook until tender to the touch. Once tender remove, drain and set aside for later use.

2. Next make your pesto. To do this add your basil, pine nuts, avocados, fresh lemon juice, garlic and olive oil into a food processor. Blend on the highest setting until smooth in consistency.

3. Season this mixture with a touch of salt and pepper.

4. Place your pasta into a large sized bowl and pour your pesto over the top. Toss well to combine.

5. Add in your tomatoes and toss again.

6. Serve with a garnish of basil and enjoy right away.

Classic Caesar Salad

There is really no other dish that is as classic as this one. For the tastiest results I highly recommend adding in some tofu of Vegan style chicken strips to make it truly delicious.

Makes: 6 to 8 Servings

Total Prep Time: 15 Minutes

Ingredients for Your Salad:

- 2 to 3 Heads of Lettuce, Romaine Variety
- 2 Tbsp. of Capers, Small in Size and Drained

Ingredients for Your Dressing:

- 1/3 Cup of Mayonnaise, Vegan Style
- 1 tsp. of Syrup, Brown Rice Variety
- 1 Tbsp. of Worcestershire Sauce, Vegan Style
- 2 Tbsp. of Lemon Juice, Fresh
- 5 Cloves of Garlic, Roasted
- ¼ Cup of Walnuts, Lightly Toasted
- ¼ Cup of Almonds, Lightly Toasted
- 2 tsp. of Yeast Flakes, Nutritional Variety
- 2 tsp. of Miso Paste, Light
- ½ tsp. of Sea Salt, For Taste
- ¼ tsp. of Black Pepper, For Taste

Ingredients for Your Croutons:

- 4 Slices of Spelt Bread
- 1 Tbsp. of Oil, Neutral Tasting Variety
- 1 tsp. of Syrup, Brown Rice Variety
- ¼ tsp. of Sea Salt, For Taste
- ¼ tsp. of Black Pepper, For Taste
- ½ tsp. of Paprika
- ¼ tsp. of Chili, Powdered Variety
- ¼ tsp. of Garlic, Powdered Variety
- ½ tsp. of Oregano, Dried

Directions:

1. First place all of your ingredients for your salad into a large sized bowl and toss thoroughly to combine. Set aside for later use.
2. Next make your dressing. To do this add your favorite mayo, rice syrup, Worcestershire sauce, fresh lemon juice, roasted garlic and remaining ingredients for your dressing into a food processor. Blend on the highest setting until creamy in smooth in consistency.
3. Remove your dressing and cover with some plastic wrap. Place into your fridge to chill for the next 30 minutes or until you are ready to use it.
4. Then make your croutons. To do this first preheat your oven to 375 degrees.
5. While your oven is heating up cut your bread into small sized pieces. Place into a large sized bowl.
6. Add in your oil, rice syrup, salt, pepper, paprika, powdered chili, powdered garlic and oregano into this bowl and toss thoroughly to coat.

7. Place this bread cubes onto a large sized ungreased baking sheet. Place into your oven to bake for the next 10 to 12 minutes or until your croutons are crispy to the touch. Remove and allow to cool slightly before using.

8. Add your croutons and dressing to your salad green and toss thoroughly to combine. Serve whenever you are ready and enjoy.

Homemade Creamy Tomato Soup

Here is a creamy and absolutely filling soup recipe that every Vegan in your household is going to be begging you for. For the tastiest results serve this dish with your favorite bread for dipping.

Makes: 6 Servings

Total Prep Time: 35 Minutes

Ingredients:

- 2 Tbsp. of Butter, Non Dairy Variety
- 1 Tbsp. of Flour, Whole Wheat Variety

- 1 Onion, Medium in Size and Chopped Finely
- 2 Cloves of Garlic, Finely Chopped
- 2 Cups of Tomatoes, Cherry Variety and Fresh
- 1, 15 Ounce Can of Tomatoes, Finely Diced
- 4 Cups of Vegetable Broth, Low in Sodium
- 1 Russet Potato, Large in Size and Finely Diced
- ¾ tsp. of Sea Salt, For Taste
- ½ tsp. of Black Pepper, For Taste
- ½ tsp. of Cinnamon, Ground Variety
- 1 Tbsp. of Lemon Juice, Fresh
- 1 Tbsp. of Agave Nectar
- ¼ Cup of Soy Creamer
- Some Croutons, For Topping

Directions:

1. Preheat a large sized pot over medium heat. Once it is hot enough add in your butter, flour, onions and garlic. Cook over

medium heat for the next 4 minutes or until slightly brown in color.

2. After this time add in your canned tomatoes and fresh tomatoes. Continue to cook for the next 2 minutes.

3. After this time add in your broth, potatoes, dash of salt, dash of pepper and cinnamon.

4. Reduce the heat to low and allow to cook at a simmer for the next 20 minutes or until your potatoes are tender to the touch.

5. After this time add in your fresh lemon juice, creamer and agave.

6. Pour into your blender and blend on the highest setting until smooth in consistency.

7. Pour back into your pot and season with a dash of salt and pepper. Heat over medium heat until piping hot. Remove and serve while still hot. Enjoy.

Hawaiian Style Sloppy Joes

Here is an easy and sweet tasting lunch or dinner dish that I guarantee even the pickiest eaters in your household are going to love. Don't hesitate to top these sandwiches with your favorite toppings to make it truly unique.

Makes: 4 Servings

Total Prep Time: 45 Minutes

Ingredients:
- 2 Tbsp. of Olive Oil, Extra Virgin Variety
- 1 Onion, Finely Chopped
- 1 Green Bell Pepper, Finely Chopped
- 8 Ounces of Mushrooms, Cremini Variety, Trimmed and Pulsed
- 2 Cloves of Garlic, Minced
- ½ tsp. of Sea Salt, For Taste
- ¼ tsp. of Red Pepper, Crushed
- 1, 15 Ounce Can of Lentils, Rinsed and Drained
- 1, 14 Ounce Can of Tomato Sauce
- ¼ Cup of Soy Sauce
- ¼ Cup of Brown Sugar, Light and Packed

- 1 Tbsp. of Vinegar, Apple Cider Variety and White
- 1 Cup of Pineapple, Fresh and Finely Chopped
- 6 Buns, Whole Wheat Variety

Directions:

1. First use a large sized pot and set it over medium to high heat. Once it is hot enough add in your oil, onions and green peppers. Cook for the next couple of minutes or until your veggies are soft to the touch.

2. Add in your mushrooms and continue to cook for an additional 8 to 10 minutes or until your mushrooms are soft to the touch.

3. After this time add in your garlic, dash of salt and red peppers. Cook for another 5 minutes.

4. Add in your lentils, tomato sauce, favorite soy sauce, brown sugar, vinegar and fresh pineapple. Stir thoroughly to combine.

5. Reduce the heat to low and allow your mixture to simmer for the next 10 to 15 minutes.

6. After this time remove from heat and allow to sit for the next 5 minutes before serving.

Winter Style White Bean Salad

This is a salad recipe that you can enjoy if you are looking to boost the amount of protein you are taking in. Easy to make it is a great tasting salad recipe to enjoy on a cold winter's night.

Makes: 4 Servings

Total Prep Time: 15 Minutes

Ingredients for Your Salad:

- 1, 2 Pound Pumpkin, Peeled and Cut into Small Sized Cubes
- 4 Cups of Cannellini Beans, Drained and Rinsed
- 1 Red Onion, Medium in Size, Peeled and Finely Diced
- Dash of Salt and Pepper, For Taste

Ingredients for Your Cilantro Pesto:

- 2 Cups of Cilantro, Packed, Freshly and Chopped Roughly
- ¼ Cup of Sunflower Seeds, Lightly Toasted and Optional
- 1 Jalapeno Pepper, Chopped Coarsely
- 4 Cloves of Garlic, Peeled and Finely Chopped
- 1 Lime, Zest and Juice Only
- Dash of Salt, For Taste
- ½ Pack of Tofu, Extra Firm and Silk Variety
- ¼ Cup of Yeast, Optional

Directions:

1. The first thing that you will want to do is steam your pumpkin in a steamer basket for the next 10 to 12 minutes or until it is tender to the touch. Once tender drain and rinsed under some running water until cool to the touch.

2. Add your pumpkin into a medium sized bowl along with your onions, beans, pesto and dash of salt and pepper. Stir thoroughly until evenly mixed.

3. Next make your cilantro pesto. To do this combine all of your ingredients for your pesto in a food processor. Blend on the highest setting until smooth and creamy in consistency.

4. Add your pumpkin salad and pesto into a large sized bowl. Toss thoroughly to coat and serve whenever you are ready. Enjoy.

Hearty Portobello Mushroom Burgers

If you are a huge fan of burgers but have been looking for a healthy vegan alternative, then this is the perfect dish for you. It is incredibly hearty and filling, making it one of those recipes I know you are going to fall in love with.

Makes: 4 Servings

Total Prep Time: 2 Hours and 35 Minutes

Ingredients:

- 2 Tbsp. of Vinegar, Balsamic Variety
- 2 Tbsp. of Vinegar, Red Wine Variety
- 1 Tbsp. of Garlic, Minced
- 2 Tbsp. of Soy Sauce, Your Favorite Kind
- 2 tsp. of Oil, Vegetable Variety

- Dash of Salt, For Taste
- 4 Mushrooms, Portobello Variety, Caps Only and Gills Removed
- Burger Buns, Your Favorite Kind

Directions:

1. Whisk together your balsamic vinegar, red wine vinegar, minced garlic, favorite soy sauce, vegetable oil and dash of salt in a medium sized bowl until evenly mixed.

2. Poke a few holes into each of your mushrooms and set into a container with the top side facing down.

3. Pour your marinade over your mushrooms and turn over lightly. Allow to marinate for the next 2 hours.

4. Next preheat your grill to medium heat. Once it is hot enough add your mushrooms onto it and grill for the next 5 minutes. Flip and continue to grill for an additional 5 minutes.

5. Remove and place onto your burger buns. Serve with your favorite toppings and enjoy.

Mongolian Style BBQ Seitan

Here is a delicious BBQ dish that you are going to love to enjoy nearly every day of the week. Packed full of authentic barbecue flavor, even the pickiest eaters in your household won't be able to resist it.

Makes: 4 Servings
Total Prep Time: 25 Minutes
Ingredients:
- ¼ Cup of Hoisin Sauce
- ¼ Cup of Water, Warm
- 1 Tbsp. of Soy Sauce, Your Favorite Kind
- 1 Tbsp. of Agave
- 1 tsp. of Lemon Juice, Fresh
- 1 to 2 tsp of Chili and Garlic Sauce
- 2 Tbsp. of Oil, Canola Variety
- 8 Ounces of Mushroom, Shiitake, Stemmed and Thinly Sliced
- 8 Ounces of Seitan, Cut into Thin Strips
- 2 tsp. of Ginger, Freshly Grated

- 1/8 tsp. of Cinnamon, Ground Variety
- 1/8 tsp. of Cloves, Ground Variety
- 4 Ounces of Snow Peas, with Strings Removed
- 2 Scallions, Trimmed and Sliced Thinly
- ¼ Cup of Cilantro, Fresh and Roughly Chopped
- 2 Cups of Rice, Fully Cooked and for Serving

Directions:

1. Use a small sized bowl and make your sauce. To do this add in your hoisin sauce, warm water, favorite soy sauce, agave, fresh lemon juice and chili and garlic sauce. Stir thoroughly to combine.

2. Next use a large sized skillet and add in your oil. Heat over medium to high heat. Once it is hot enough add in your mushrooms and seitan. Cook until light brown in color.

3. Then add in your ginger, cinnamon and ground cloves. Stir thoroughly to combine and allow to cook for the next 8 minutes.

4. Add in your sauce and snow peas.

5. Reduce the heat to low and allow to cook until your sauce is thick in consistency.

6. Once thick remove from heat and add in your scallions and cilantro. Stir to combine and serve over a bed of rice. Enjoy whenever you are ready.

Tasty Mushroom Stroganoff

If you are looking for a filling meal that the entire family will enjoy, then this is the perfect dish for you to make. It is so delicious I guarantee the entire family will be begging you for more.

Makes: 4 Servings

Total Prep Time: 40 Minutes

Ingredients:

- 2 Shallots, Large in Size, Peeled and Minced
- 8 Cloves of Garlic, Peeled and Minced
- 2 tsp. of Thyme, Minced
- Dash of Salt and Pepper, For Taste
- 1 tsp. of Rosemary, Minced

- 1 Pound of Mushrooms, Portobello Variety, Stemmed and Cut into Large Sized Pieces
- 1 Ounce of Mushrooms, Porcini Variety, Soaked and Chopped Roughly
- ½ Cup of White Wine, Dry Variety
- 1 Pound of Fettucine, Fully Cooked and Warm
- Some Parsley, Fresh and Chopped Roughly

Ingredients for Your Tofu Sour Cream:
- 1, 12 Ounce Pack of Tofu, Extra Firm and Drained
- 1 Tbsp. of Lemon Juice, Fresh
- 1 Tbsp. of Vinegar, Red Wine Variety

Directions:

1. Place your shallots into a large sized skillet and set over medium heat. Cook for the next 8 minutes before adding in your water, garlic and thyme. Continue to cook for an additional minute.

2. Add in your dash of salt and pepper, rosemary and mushrooms. Continue to

cook for another 10 minutes, making sure to stir thoroughly as it cooks.

3. Add in your porcini mushrooms, wine and soaking liquid. Stir to combine and reduce the heat to low or medium. Cook for another 20 minutes.

4. Stir in to your sour cream and cooked noodles. Remove from heat and toss thoroughly to combine. Garnish with some fresh parsley.

5. Next make your tofu sour cream. To do this combine all of your ingredients for your cream into a blender. Blend on the highest setting until smooth and creamy in consistency. Season with some salt and serve with your stroganoff. Enjoy.

Tempeh Chimichurri

This is a delicious vegan style recipe that you are going to love especially if you are looking for something more on the light side. Serve this with your favorite steamed veggies for the tastiest results.

Makes: 6 Servings

Total Prep Time: 30 Minutes

Ingredients:

- 8 Ounces of Tempeh, Thin Slabs and Thinly Sliced

Ingredients for Your Chimichurri:

- 4 Cloves of Garlic, Minced
- 1 Cup of Cilantro, Fresh and Packed Loosely
- 1 tsp. of Oregano, Dried
- ¼ Cup of Vinegar, Red Wine Variety
- 2 Tbsp. of Olive Oil, Extra Virgin Variety
- ½ tsp. of Red Pepper Flakes
- ½ tsp. of Salt, For Taste
- ¾ Cup of Vegetable Broth, Homemade Preferable
- 1 Tbsp. of Soy Sauce, Your Favorite Kind

Directions:

1. The first thing that you will want to do is steam your tempeh for at least 10 minutes.

2. While your tempeh is steaming make your chimichurri. To do this add all of your

ingredients for your chimichurri into a blender and blend on the highest setting until smooth in consistency.

3. Place your steamed tempeh onto a large sized plate. Add at least half a cup of your chimichurri into a bowl along with your soy sauce. Stir thoroughly to combine. Reserve your remaining chimichurri.

4. Pour your chimichurri mixture over the top of your tempeh and allow to sit for at least one hour.

5. Then preheat a large sized pan over medium to high heat. Add in a thin layer of oil and once it is hot enough add in your tempeh and cook for at least 3 minutes on all sides.

6. Serve with your reserved chimichurri drizzled over the top and enjoy.

Classic Penne Marinara

This is one of my all-time favorite vegan recipes and once you get a taste of it yourself I know it will become one of your favorites as well. Feel free to serve this dish up with your favorite bread for the tastiest results.

Makes: 2 Servings

Total Prep Time: 15 Minutes

Ingredients:

- 3 Cups of Penne Pasta, Whole Grain Variety
- 2 Tbsp. of Olive Oil, Extra Virgin Variety
- 1 Onion, Small in Size and Finely Chopped
- 1 Cup of Water, Cold
- 1 Cup of Tomato Paste
- 4 Cloves of Garlic, Finely Diced
- ¼ tsp. of Black Pepper, For Taste
- 1 tsp. of Salt, For Taste
- ¼ Cup of Basil, Fresh and Finely Diced

Directions:

1. The first thing that you will want to do is cook your pasta according to the directions on the package. Once cooked, drain and set aside for later use.

2. Next make your sauce. To do this add your onions into a large sized skillet with some olive oil placed over medium heat. Cook until your onions are transparent.

3. Then add in your tomato paste, garlic, dash of salt, dash of pepper and fresh basil. Stir thoroughly to combine.

4. Add in your water slowly, making sure to stir thoroughly the entire time.

5. Cover and allow to simmer at low heat for the next 10 minutes. Make sure to stir occasionally.

6. Remove from heat and pour your sauce over your cooked pasta. Garnish with some fresh basil and enjoy.

Hearty Shepherd's Pie

Here is another taste dinner recipe that you are going to want to make for your friends and family. It is so tasty I guarantee that your family will want to come back for seconds.

Makes: 6 Servings

Total Prep Time: 1 Hour and 5 Minutes

Ingredients for Your Mashed Potato Layer:

- 5 Russet Potatoes, Peeled and Cut into Small Sized Cubes
- ½ Cup of Mayonnaise, Vegan Variety
- ½ Cup of Milk, Soy Variety
- ¼ Cup of Olive Oil, Extra Virgin Variety
- 3 Tbsp. of Cream Cheese, Vegan Variety
- 2 tsp. of Salt, For Taste

Ingredients for Your Bottom Layer:

- 1 Tbsp. of Oil, Vegetable Variety
- 1 Onion, Yellow in Color and Finely Chopped
- 2 Carrots, Fresh and Finely Chopped
- ½ Cup of Peas, Frozen Variety
- 3 Stalks of Celery, Freshly Chopped
- 1 Tomato, Fresh and Finely Chopped
- 1 tsp. of Italian Seasoning
- 1 Clove of Garlic, Minced and for Taste
- Dash of Black Pepper, For Taste
- 1, 14 Ounce Pack of Beef, Vegetarian variety, Lean and Ground

- ½ Cup of Cheese, Soy Variety and Finely Shredded

Directions:

1. First place your potatoes into a large sized pot and cover with some water. Set over medium to high heat and bring to a boil. Once boiling reduce the heat to low and allow your potatoes to boil for the next 25 minutes or until they are tender to the touch. After this time drain and set aside for later use.

2. Add your potatoes into a large sized bowl along with your mayonnaise, milk, olive oil, cream cheese and dash of salt. Mash thoroughly using a potato masher until smooth and fluffy in consistency. Set aside for later use.

3. Next preheat your oven to 400 degrees. While your oven is heating up spray a large sized baking dish with a generous amount of cooking spray.

4. Next heat up a large sized skillet over medium heat. Add in your oil and add in your onions, fresh carrots, fresh tomatoes,

fresh celery and frozen peas. Cook for the next 10 minutes before stirring in your Italian seasoning, garlic and dash of pepper.

5. Reduce the heat to low and add in your vegetarian beef. Continue to cook for the next 5 minutes or until piping hot.

6. Spread your beef mixture into the bottom of your baking dish. Top off with your mashed potatoes and smooth out into an even layer. Top off with your cheese.

7. Place into your oven to bake for the next 20 minutes or until slightly brown in color. Remove and serve right away.

Decadent Chocolate and Strawberry

Shortcake Cupcakes

Just as the name implies this is one dish that you will want to make whenever you need to satisfy your strongest sweet tooth. These cupcakes are so sweet I know you won't be able to get enough of it.

Makes: 6 Servings

Total Prep Time: 35 Minutes

Ingredients for Your Chocolate Cupcakes:

- 1 ½ Cups of Flour, All Purpose Variety
- 1 Cup of Sugar
- 1/3 Cup of Cocoa Powder, Unsweetened Variety
- 1 tsp. of Baker's Style Baking Soda
- ½ tsp. of Salt, For Taste
- 1 Cup of Milk, Coconut Variety
- ½ Cup of Oil, Canola Variety
- 2 Tbsp. of Vinegar, Apple Cider Variety
- 2 tsp. of Vanilla, Pure

Ingredients for Your Frosting:

- 1 Cup of Shortening, Vegetable Variety
- 3 Cups of Sugar, Powdered Variety
- 1 tsp. of Vanilla, Pure
- 2 to 5 Tbsp. of Milk, Soy Variety

Ingredients for Your Garnish:

- 1 ½ Cups of Strawberries, Fresh and Thinly Sliced
- Dash of Sugar, Powdered Variety

Directions:

1. The first thing that you will want to do is make your cupcakes. To do this first preheat your oven to 350 degrees. While your oven is heating up line two cupcake pans with cupcake liners.
2. Then use a large sized bowl and add in your flour, white sugar, cocoa, baker's style baking soda and dash of salt. Whisk thoroughly to combine.
3. Add in your separate bowl and add in your coffee, oil, vanilla and vinegar. Whisk thoroughly to combine and pour into your dry mixture. Stir again to combine.
4. Fill your cupcake liners at least 2/3 of the way full with your batter.
5. Place into your oven to bake for at least 16 to 18 minutes or until your cupcakes are completely baked through. Remove and allow your cupcakes to cool completely.
6. Next make your frosting. To do this place your shortening into a large sized bowl. Use an electric mixer and beat until smooth in consistency.

7. Then add in your sugar, pure vanilla and milk. Continue to beat until smooth in consistency and fluffy in texture.

8. Next assemble your cupcakes. To do this slather your cupcakes with your frosting and sliced strawberries. Dust with some powdered sugar and serve whenever you are ready.

Decadent Peanut Butter Bonbons

Here is yet another sweet tasting dessert dish that you can make whenever you want to make a sweet treat for your friends and family. Make these and wrap them to make tasty gifts.

Makes: 16 to 20 Servings
Total Prep Time: 30 Minutes
Ingredients:
- ¼ Cup of Butter, Non Dairy Variety
- 1 ½ Cups of Sugar, Powdered Variety
- 1 Cup of Peanut Butter, Smooth Variety

- 1 Cup of Bread Crumbs, Organic and Unseasoned Variety
- ¼ tsp. of Cinnamon, Ground Variety
- ¼ tsp. of Sea Salt, For Taste
- 1 tsp. of Vanilla, Pure
- 1, 12 Ounce Pack of Chocolate Chips, Vegan Variety and Dark in Color
- 1 Tbsp. of Oil, Neutral Tasting Variety
- ¼ Cup of Peanuts, Ground Variety

Directions:

1. Next use a large sized bowl and add in your butter, powdered sugar, smooth peanut butter, bread crumbs, dash of cinnamon, salt and pure vanilla. Use an electric mixer and blend until smooth in consistency.

2. Roll your mixture into small sized bowl and place onto an ungreased cookie sheet lined with some parchment paper. Place into your freezer to freeze for the next 20 minutes.

3. Next create a double boiler. Add in your chocolate chips and cook over medium heat until your chocolate is completely

melted. Add in your oil and whisk thoroughly until smooth in consistency.

4. Remove your balls from your freezer and dip each ball into your chocolate.

5. Place your balls back onto your cookie sheet and place back into your freezer to freeze up. Remove and allow to sit for 5 minutes prior to serving.

Zesty Lemon Bars

Last we have this great tasting dessert recipe that you won't be able to resist. These bars are the perfect dessert dish to enjoy after having a full and satisfying vegan meal.

Makes: 8 Servings

Total Prep Time: 1 Hour and 5 Minutes

Ingredients for Your Crust:
- ½ Cup of Butter, Non Dairy Variety and Soft
- ¼ Cup of Sugar, Confectioner's Variety
- 1 Cup of Flour, All Purpose Variety

Ingredients for Your Filling:
- ½ Cup of Tofu, Silk Variety

- 1 Cup of Sugar, Granulated Variety
- 2 Lemons, Zest Only
- 1/3 Cup of Lemon Juice, Fresh
- 2 Tbsp. of Flour, All Purpose Variety
- 2 Tbsp. of Cornstarch
- Dash of Sugar, Confectioner's Variety and Sifted

Directions:

1. The first thing that you will want to do is preheat your oven to 350 degrees. While your oven is heating up grease a large sized baking pan with some canola oil and sprinkle some flour into it.

2. Next make your crust. To do this first add your butter and confectioner's sugar into a large sized bowl and cream together until fluffy in consistency.

3. Add in your flour and continue to beat with an electric mixer until a dough begins to form.

4. Place your crust into the bottom of your prepared pan. Place into your oven to bake for the next 20 minutes or until light brown in color. After this time remove

your crust from your oven and allow to cool on a wire rack.

5. Then make your filling. To do this first add your tofu into a food processor. Blend on the highest setting until smooth in consistency. Add in your fresh lemon zest, fresh lemon juice, flour and cornstarch. Blend again to combine.

6. Pour your freshly made filling into your crust and place back into your oven to bake for the next 30 minutes or until it is set to the touch.

7. After this time remove from your oven and set aside to cool. Dust with your confectioner's sugar before serving. Enjoy.

Conclusion

So, there you have it!
Hopefully by the end of this book you have learned what it takes to live a truly vegan lifestyle. I hope that by the end of this

book you have learned not only how to make some of the most delicious Vegan meals you will ever come across, but I also hope that you have learned what ingredients you should use that are considered to be Vegan friendly.

So, what is next for you?

The next step for you to take is to begin making all of the recipes you have found in this book. Once you have done that it is time for you to begin looking for other vegan friendly recipes out there until you are able to make and enjoy vegan meals every day of the week.

Good luck!

About the Author

Fred Dowd is author of several cookbooks on Vegan diet. He has written research papers on the topic and currently lives in California.

www.ingramcontent.com/pod-product-compliance
Lightning Source LLC
LaVergne TN
LVHW011949070526
838202LV00054B/4864